Athlete's foot no more

Thank you for buying my book. The advice contained herein is completely unbiased, as my only income is from the sale of this information and not driven by the hope of earning a commission or other financial gain from the sale of any product.

Permit me to start by explaining why I developed this remedy.

A few years ago, I had an attack of athlete's foot which resisted multiple attempts to eradicate despite using a variety of non prescription creams and powders. I also tried soaking my feet in salted water with no noticeable improvement.

For many years I have tried to remedy minor ailments myself, so it was with great reluctance and in desperation, due to the fact that I had an open wound caused by the infection which was getting deeper, that I visited our doctor.

Our doctor agreed that it was in fact athlete's foot and initially prescribed a cream that was available without a prescription. However, when I pointed out that I had already used this cream to little effect he changed the prescription to a different cream which was only available with a prescription.
This I duly used, as per the instructions, continuing the treatment for 10 days after the athlete's foot appeared to have been eliminated and the skin had healed.

Some weeks later the itching started again and once more I applied the prescribed cream until the skin was healed, continuing as recommended for an additional 10 days.

Several weeks later the itching returned. Yet again, I applied the prescribed cream until the skin was healed, continuing as recommended for another period of 10 days.

By now I was getting pretty fed up with this not so 'merry-go-round' and resolved to find an alternative, hopefully better, solution.

This frustrating roundabout of infection, treatment, infection, treatment led me to start thinking about possible alternatives. I know that the fungus and bacteria combination that causes athlete's foot does not like dry conditions or contact with moving air, however the infection persisted, even during the warmer months when I was able to wear sandals.

I am not going to pull any punches here. The ailment commonly known as athlete's foot causes itching and pain for a very simple reason.
Athlete's foot is a combination of fungus and bacteria that are quite literally eating you alive!

Therefore it is best not to dismiss it as a minor problem and to take no action in the hopes that it will clear up of its own accord. **It will not.**

You can choose to follow my early failed attempts to rid your feet of the infection or you can opt to follow the simple and highly effective remedy that I have since devised.

As you will read later on, I was already aware that ozone is a powerful disinfectant, however, I did not know if I could use it to kill the infection that causes athlete's foot, nor did I have any idea as to how I would be able to use ozone for this particular application.

According to my research, ozone is equally as lethal to micro-organisms as chlorine, that is to say it kills 99.99% of all known germs. Importantly, it kills in a fraction of the time taken by chlorine and is much safer to use. I certainly would not want to use chlorine on my skin at a strong enough concentration for it to be effective. In order to create ozone at home I ordered an ozone generator and experimented, using myself as a human 'guinea pig'.

Once the ozone generator had been delivered and unpacked, I found it very simple to operate and wasted no time putting it into service.

My initial trials involved using a foot bath with the ozone bubbling into the water. This proved to be a failure as it did not eliminate the infection.
I know that the micro-organisms that cause athlete's foot do not like dry conditions, therefore I resolved to find a way of applying the ozone without using water.

I found that if I applied the ozone and air mixture straight from the open end of the flexible tubing attached to the ozone generator, this proved to be highly effective. The death of the infectious fungus and bacteria combination that caused my athlete's foot was rapid and the skin returned to its normal appearance much more quickly than it had done previously using the prescription cream.

It is now 3 or 4 years since I developed this method and during this time I have had several less serious infections and one more serious attack involving several toe joints, all of which have been successfully and rapidly remedied using ozone.

In order to benefit from this highly effective drug-free treatment that can easily be administered at home, you need to purchase an '**Air and Water Ozone Generator**'. This can be purchased on the internet from around £30 and has a built-in timer, and must be supplied with a length of silicone tubing. This is the only type of tubing that is ozone resistant.

There are numerous models of ozone generators on the market, however I have specified **Air and Water** as this is the only type that allows the user to direct the ozone to where it is needed, in this case between the toes. Verify that your chosen model is supplied with a length of tubing and a diffuser before placing your order.

It is important that you should know that an ozone generator's output is rated in milligrams per hour, or, in the case of more powerful models, grams per hour. I opted for a unit rated at 600 milligrams per hour. This is the rating that I recommend that you should purchase as my own experience has shown that this is adequate for facilitating the rapid destruction of the infection.

Ozone generators use electrical energy to convert some of the oxygen in the air into ozone and a built-in pump delivers the ozone enriched air via the flexible tube to where it is required.

My first experiment using dry ozone to kill the micro-organisms involved just one toe joint and was simply a matter of holding the flexible tube, gripping it lightly with the toes on each side of the infected joint. I put the open end of the tube to face the infected joint in order to bathe the area with ozone. I found that a daily, five minute treatment worked well for a relatively mild infection. Please note that a number of daily treatments may be required to ensure complete elimination of the infection.

A later infection, involving several joints, required me to develop a more efficient system, as I quickly realised that a more widespread infection required a different approach. I was not willing to devote the amount of time that would have been required to treat each joint individually. I tried several options and I concluded that a simple polythene food bag was an inexpensive and effective way of bathing the entire infected area with ozone. The polythene bag can be used multiple times, as the interior of the bag will be sterilised with each use. Needless to say, the bag should be large enough to cover your entire foot.

The method that I have found works well is to hold the open end of the flexible tube between any pair of toes, this time with the open end facing forward (i.e. away from your toe joints) with the tube running along the length of your foot.

Now place the polythene bag over your foot and gather the excess width, so that the open end of the bag is a snug fit around your foot or your ankle depending on
the size of your bag. You can simply hold the excess polythene underneath your foot so that the weight of your foot holds the bag in place. This ensures that most of the ozone is retained in the bag where it is needed, in order for it to have the desired effect.

Having secured the open end of the bag around my foot, I gently squeeze the sealed end in order to expel as much air as possible. As the bag inflates during the treatment, I know that the concentration of ozone is maximized around the toes. Now simply switch on your ozone generator for 5 minutes or more depending on the level of infection that you are treating, occasionally spreading your toes to ensure that the ozone can make contact with all of the infected skin.

There are numerous options for closing the open end of the bag. A length of string, a shoe lace, a length of ribbon just to mention a few. There is also the modern alternative of a hook and loop ribbon. This is the type of ribbon that has one side with hooks and the other side with loops, and readily clings to itself. After cutting a suitable length, pass this around your foot at the point where you want to close the bag and gently press the two opposing sides together. This eliminates tying and untying knots and is useful to those who find it a challenge to reach down to their feet.

For severely infected feet, a longer period of treatment may be required, perhaps as much as 15 minutes per foot. In this case, I suggest starting with a daily, or even better, twice daily (morning and evening) routine and gradually reducing to daily and then alternate days once you are confident that the healing process is well under way.

As per the recommendations provided with pharmaceutical treatments, it may be a wise option to continue the ozone treatments for a few days after your skin appears to have returned to normal, perhaps at the reduced time of five minutes once a day.

It is important to realise that although the ozone **will** quickly kill the micro-organisms causing the infection, the process of healing will take longer. The only way that you can be sure that the treatments have been effective is when you see healthy new skin between your toes. It is a fact that the skin healing takes longer than the fungus killing process. For this reason it can be tricky to judge when to stop the treatment, however as the ozone appears to have no harmful side effects on one's feet I recommend that you continue until you feel confident that the treatment has completely eliminated the infection.

Continuing the treatment for longer will have the added advantage of keeping the wound area sterile, which can only help to speed up the healing process.

NOTE. My research indicates that ozone is **not** absorbed through the skin.

I have absolute confidence in the ability of ozone to kill micro-organisms.
One of the great advantages of ozone is that it attacks and kills both the fungus and the associated bacteria in a way that denies them any possibility of developing a resistant strain. Therefore, no matter how many times the athlete's foot returns you will always be able to rely on ozone to return your feet to good health.

In the unlikely event that you do not achieve the desired outcome, the first thing to consider is whether the ozone is actually able to contact the infected area. For example, if the infection is located under the toe, it is most likely to be in the area where the skin folds in such a way that denies the ozone any possibility of making contact.
You can easily demonstrate this to yourself by the simple action of folding a finger. When your finger is folded there is an area of skin that disappears from view. Exactly the same can happen with your toes and will prevent the ozone from accessing the infected area.

Holding the toe straight for the duration of the treatment is not a realistic option. However, it is simple enough to repeatedly straighten your toes during the time that you are treating the infection.

If for any reason you are unable to straighten your toes, do not despair, as I have found that placing the air stone directly under the infected joint works well. Needless to say, the air stone needs to be connected to the ozone generator by means of the flexible tubing. As the air stone allows the ozone to escape in all directions it is, as previously described, helpful to wrap the area being treated with polythene so that as much of the ozone as possible is retained where it is needed.

When you purchase your ozone generator you may find that the instructions state different treatment times to those shown above. The instructions provided with my ozone generator quote '20 to 30 minutes for hands and feet' with no further guidance. The times that I have listed above are those that have worked for me.

The times that I have mentioned above should be considered merely as guidance. You may need to experiment and adapt those times in order to discover what suits your own needs and requirements.

 It really is a simple matter of getting started and in the event that you do not see any improvement after several days, then simply increase the length and or frequency of your treatment sessions, at the same time ensuring that the ozone can make contact with all the areas that are infected.

Unless you are very fortunate, the athlete's foot may well return at a later date. If this happens, simply repeat the above process, bearing in mind that the sooner you start the treatment, the shorter the duration of treatment will be, both in terms of the number of individual treatments and the time required for each treatment.
It has been my experience that if I act at the very first sign of an irritation, then a single treatment of just five minutes usually suffices.

Ozone is a fast and effective treatment that compares very favourably with creams that may require up to two months to kill an infection.

In order to reduce the possibility of a repeat infection, it is a good idea to sterilize the insides of your footwear. The most effective way to do this is with an ultraviolet shoe steriliser, which generates a small amount of ozone. A shoe steriliser can be purchased for about £30.
Do not be tempted to use the ultraviolet shoe sterilizer to treat any skin conditions. There is a considerable risk of burning your skin and ultraviolet is extremely damaging to eyes. Not only human eyes!

When sterilising shoes with ultraviolet light, take precautions to ensure the safety of children and pets.

Since purchasing and using an ultraviolet shoe steriliser I have enjoyed a reduction of repeat infections of athlete's foot to almost zero. An additional advantage is that leather shoes that have been sterilised will regain that new, just out of the box, smell of leather.

I absolutely **do not** recommend using your ozone generator to sterilise your shoes. Despite ozone being an obvious choice for this task as it is very effective as a footwear sterilizer it is also VERY aggressive towards SOME synthetic materials. One industrial use for ozone that I am aware of, is accelerated age testing of certain rubber products. You can easily demonstrate this to yourself by stretching an elastic band around your foot on the **outside** of the polythene bag whilst you are killing the infection with ozone. In my experience the elastic band will decay and fall apart in a few minutes, and that, in case you are wondering, is why I have not suggested that you use an elastic band to hold the polythene bag in place, even though the use of an elastic band would seem to be a prime candidate for this task.

For those readers who have no experience of ozone I include the following information.

Ozone is entirely natural in the upper atmosphere where it helps to protect our planet from the sun's harmful levels of ultraviolet radiation.

One of the ways that ozone is created in nature is by lightning, however, it can be produced in a home environment by electricity using a system known as corona discharge. A corona discharge requires the generation of a high voltage. The resulting controlled discharge of the high voltage converts some of the oxygen (O2) in the air into ozone (O3).

When you purchase your ozone generator, the unit that creates the high voltage will be an integral part of the generator. Do not be alarmed by the fact that high voltage is used as it is actually much less dangerous than the electricity that we use on a daily basis and take for granted in our homes and at work!

In order to clarify the preceding statement I need to get a bit technical. Electricity is referenced in two main ways, voltage and current. Current is measured in amperes or amps. A relatively low voltage coupled with a high current is far more dangerous than the high voltage used in an ozone generator which has almost zero current.

The danger to life occurs when the voltage and the current are present together at sufficient levels, such as is the case with our household electricity supply. In order to illustrate the difference, I will recount two actual events that, I hope, will enable you to better understand the difference.
The first event involving low voltage and high current occurred during the Second World War, when my father was a young man. He accidentally dropped a spanner onto a 24 volt lorry battery. The spanner was instantly welded onto the 2 battery terminals and within a matter of seconds was glowing red-hot. This was as a direct result of the very high current available.
The second event occurred, well after the end of the war, in my father's television repair workshop. One of his engineers was investigating a working television when his arm got too close to the point on the cathode ray tube where the 25,000 volts is injected. He was completely unaware that the high voltage was arcing onto his arm until he was informed by another engineer. If that had been 250 volts but at a higher current, he would most certainly have been a great deal more than aware!

I hope that I have put your mind at rest and have assured you that the high voltage involved in the production of ozone is both contained and safe and not a cause for concern. In any case, ozone generators have to be tested and certified safe for home use, as with any electrical appliance.

If you still have any doubts regarding the safety of the high voltage used, you can be further reassured by the fact that a toy for children, the plasma ball, uses the same type of high voltage to create the captive lightning effect. When you touch the ball, the 'lightning' is drawn to your finger, but there is not the slightest sensation of electricity flowing into your body.

Although the 12 volts of a car battery will not kill you, the high level of current available necessitates that a set of jump leads should be used with a great deal of care and respect.

Under normal circumstances, and at ground level, ozone is extremely unstable and quickly returns to its previous state of oxygen. However it stays as ozone for more than long enough to destroy the fungus and bacteria combination which is the cause of athlete's foot. This it does by splitting open the cell walls of the micro-organisms so that they effectively 'bleed to death'. It is this action that ensures that the micro-organisms are completely incapable of developing a resistant strain or of mutating.

A FEW EXAMPLES OF THE MANY USES FOR OZONE.

Some refrigerators now include a built-in ozone generator which extends the storage life of fresh produce by killing the micro-organisms that would otherwise cause the stored fresh produce to decay more quickly.

Have you ever wondered how bottled water stays fresh and clear? Yet another example of the ability of ozone to sterilise. Unlike chlorine it does not taint the water.

Ozone is used in high doses to sterilise some operating theatres and dentist treatment rooms (whilst not in use) and in some swimming pools. In the case of swimming pools the ozone is dissolved in the water and as a result, presents no danger, no odour and does not damage swim-wear. The fact that ozone is used on a regular basis to treat health care areas, must surely offer us a considerable level of assurance that ozone not only kills the micro-organisms, but also denies them any possibility of mutating.

Some years ago there was an unpleasant odour in one of our bedroom's following a family member having been unwell for several days.

Repeatedly airing the room proved to be completely ineffective. At the time I had an ozone generator rated at 10 grams an hour. This generator was the type used for swimming pools and therefore did not have a built-in timer. The lack of a timer meant that it was not ideally suited for the purpose of room sterilisation, for reasons that will become clear later.

Having closed the doors and windows of the bedroom I switched on the ozone generator and quickly left the room leaving the generator to run for an hour. When the hour had passed I went back into the room, switched off the generator and opened the window, all the time holding my breath until after I had left the room. The room then remained unoccupied with the window open for another hour. Had I not been able, for any reason, to air the treated room, it would have been simply a matter of switching off the generator, leaving the room, and waiting until the ozone had returned to its previous state of oxygen before reoccupying the room.

Ozone returning to its former state of oxygen is an unstoppable process that will occur completely naturally and in a relatively short space of time. The result of this treatment was astounding. The unpleasant odour had been entirely eliminated and did not return.

Do not be tempted to use a high output ozone generator in a room which is occupied. This advice also applies to any areas where there are pets.

Some further advice for those readers planning to buy a high output ozone generator as a result of reading my book.

These are readily available from around £40 for a home unit which is intended for occasional use. My research has shown that there are, in essence, three ratings available. 10, 20 and 28 grams per hour (gph). In order to assist you in making your choice, may I suggest that your choice should be governed by the size of your home. 10 gph for a modest home, 28 gph for a large home and 20 gph for those that fall in between. I chose a 28 gph model, not because we live in a large house, but because I intend to take it on holiday with me so that, in view of the current pandemic, I can sterilise anything from a hotel room to an entire holiday cottage in the least time possible.

A high power generator is basically a box containing the equipment needed to generate ozone and a fan to ensure that the ozone is distributed around the entire room.
Make sure that your chosen generator is fitted with a timer, the timer normally has a maximum run time of 60 minutes. A timer is absolutely vital and will enable you to take full advantage of the ability of ozone to kill bacteria, viruses and mould. It is even capable of killing so called 'superbugs'.

The fan within the ozone generator is not very powerful. It would be of considerable benefit in terms of boosting its circulating power, to run a circulating fan in the same room during the treatment. The more the air is stirred, the greater the chances of the ozone reaching all parts of the room.

The timer will enable you to sterilise a bedroom while you are away from home. Set the generator to work for your chosen time just before leaving your home. When you return home, after a day at work, the ozone generator will have switched off on reaching the end of the time period that you have chosen. During the chosen run-time it will have sterilised your entire bedroom, provided that the time that you have selected is sufficient for the volume of the room. By the time that you return home the ozone will have retuned to its normal state of oxygen, enabling you to safely enter the room. The odour created by ozone may linger for a couple of days, however, on its own, this odour is not dangerous. Personally, I find the odour to be reassuring, as I do the smell of disinfectant.

Whilst on the subject of bedrooms, it may be helpful for you to know that ozone can also be used to sterilise the contents of your wardrobe. If you are using a high powered generator to sterilise the room it is simply a matter of leaving the wardrobe doors open. Alternatively you can use your 600mg per hour generator inside a wardrobe with the doors closed. As ozone is heavier than air it is necessary to place the generator as high as possible in the wardrobe. This requirement does not apply to a high power generator as the unit contains a fan to stir the air.

One word of caution here. **Do not** place the generator close to any garments that contain elastic or similar products as repeated use of concentrated ozone in close proximity to such garments may destroy the elasticity. Sterilising the contents of your wardrobe will have the additional benefit of removing any odours that may be present.

In order to sterilise a living room you can switch on the generator just before going to bed and in the morning, as if by magic, you will discover a fresh smelling living room, almost as if it had been redecorated and all the furniture is new.

It may be helpful for you to know that because ozone is a gas it can penetrate even the tiniest of spaces. According to my research, ozone kills micro-organisms more quickly than chlorine based products. Best of all, because it is a gas, it can sterilise more efficiently and more thoroughly than someone spending a considerable amount of time using a liquid disinfectant.

In order to sterilise a room while you are at home my advice would be, if possible, to lock the door of the room that you are sterilising and remove the key. If you cannot lock the room, then think about blocking the doorway with something moveable that will act as a reminder, for example, a chair.

This is vital if you have small children and important for everyone else. It would be easy enough for anyone, especially children, to forget and to enter the room too soon.

My advice about not entering a room where the ozone generator is working is probably a case of being over-cautious for the majority of adults.

If you were to enter the room being treated, the odour of ozone would very quickly remind you to leave the room as soon as possible with no risk to your health.

Clearly, this is not the case with children or pets, that is why I strongly advise you to ensure that they cannot gain access to a room where a high power generator is in use, or for at least an hour after the treatment time has ended.

Once again I remind you that high levels of ozone coupled with prolonged exposure can be dangerous. **DO NOT attempt to sterilise a room that is occupied or will be occupied before the ozone has had sufficient time to disperse via an open window or to return naturally to its previous and preferred state of oxygen.**

I have not offered any guidance as to the times required for the sterilisation tasks outlined above. This is because the sizes of rooms and wardrobes vary, as does the output of ozone generators. My advice is to simply get started and learn from your experiences. In the majority of cases it should not possible to over-dose.
In the event that your selected period of treatment time proves to be insufficient simply repeat the process for a longer time. When I treated our bedroom of 30 cubic metres, I used a 10gph generator for one hour.

Warning – Lung conditions. U.K. national health guidance warns against prolonged exposure to high levels of ozone. This advice is primarily aimed at people whose work involves day long exposure to ozone. Even though this criteria is not likely to be met using the treatment regime for athlete's foot outlined above, some people with lung problems, in particular asthma, may not be able to cope with the relatively small amount of ozone that escapes from the confines of the bag. If you have any doubts then I recommend that you consult a heath professional.

For those readers who want to take advantage of the incredible power of ozone but are concerned about possible lung damage, I offer the following suggestions. It may be possible to carry out the treatment outside (weather permitting) or with ample ventilation, or possibly using a circulating fan placed in the same room in order to stir the air, this will ensure that the ozone is diluted.

I actually use this method myself when using ozone for a period of treatment longer than five minutes.
Some people will barely notice the distinctive pungent odour of ozone whilst a minority may find it unacceptable.
This is not the same as the odour that we associate with the seaside.

It may be that I have developed something of a 'blind spot' when it comes to the distinctive odour of ozone.

During my childhood and up to the age of 21 my father repaired a vast number of televisions. At home and later in his shop where I chose to spend as much of my time as possible.

When I was 6 years old and Queen Elizabeth II was crowned we had the only television in our road and our living room was filled to capacity with neighbours who were eager to watch the coronation on our 9 inch, round, black and white television screen. I am telling you this so that you understand that the following relates to early models of televisions. One of the requirements for a cathode ray tube to be able to produce a picture is 25,000 volts. Needless to say the insulating products that were available at that time were somewhat primitive and leaks of such a high voltage were common and inevitably created ozone. For this reason I have experienced the odour of ozone a great many times, leading me to think that I may be slightly nose blind when it comes to the odour of ozone and that others may notice it more keenly than I do.

At this point I am including a question that has puzzled me since I was at school even though it has absolutely no relevance to the topic of this article.
As a result of my experience with these early televisions, I know for a fact that 25,000 volts can jump approximately one inch or 2.5cms. This knowledge led me to wonder how many volts might be required to generate a lightning strike. Needless to say this information is now available on the internet.

After a while of regularly using ozone in a foot bath I became so used to the odour that I got to the point where I thought that my generator was producing less ozone than previously, leading me to replace it with a new one. When the new one arrived and I was able to compare it with the original model. There was no detectable difference.

I have not made any recommendations that you should use a foot bath in conjunction with ozone to cure athlete's foot, because, quite simply it does not work! After a great many attempts I have concluded that the water in the foot bath is so shallow that the bubbles reach the surface before they have had time to dissolve. I am rather dismayed by this unfortunate fact, because, for a short time we had a swimming pool which was sanitised by ozone.

The method of injecting ozone into the water ensured that it was completely dissolved and this led to the water rapidly improving the overall health of my feet. Since selling the property, I have been unable to replicate the conditions required to dissolve the ozone and I have now abandoned these attempts.

My wife and I have used ozone on many occasions, not just on our feet but for several other applications with zero ill effects. To put your mind at rest, as I do not want you to decide not to proceed with my recommendations due to any doubts you may have regarding the use of ozone, I would like to point out the following:

Ozone generators have been sold for many years, and continue to be sold, as air odour removal appliances which would certainly imply that they are safe to use.

Whilst the majority of these appliances produce smaller quantities of ozone albeit over longer periods of time than the model that you will be using to cure athlete's foot fungus, there will be, none the less, a build-up of ozone in the area being treated which will likely exceed the quantity that escapes from the polythene bag during your short treatment time.
If these appliances posed any serious threat to human health then one can be sure that the sale of them would have been banned long ago.

I have had a question in my mind for many years concerning anal irritation, commonly referred to as 'jock itch'.

I wondered if this came about as a result of putting on my underwear. After all the first part of my body that passes through my underwear is my feet.

My question was whether it was likely or even possible that the fungus spores could be moved from my feet to the area surrounding my anus by the action of putting on my underwear.

I believe that I now have an answer to that question. Since killing the infection between my toes with ozone in combination with disinfecting my shoes using ultraviolet light, it appears that I have dramatically reduced the upwards transmission of the micro-organisms.

The fungus spores can also be moved from the feet to other parts of your body following contact with your hands. The best advice is to thoroughly wash your hands after touching your feet.

Prior to owning an ozone generator I had, on multiple occasions, used a variety of creams to remedy this particularly irritating infection. I had even resorted to sitting in a shallow bath of salty water.

In view of the fact that I would rather not use my fingers to apply cream to this not very hygienic area of my body, I decided to try and find a way of using ozone. Unlike the method that I used for my feet a polythene bag was clearly a non starter.

Eventually I came up with the idea of using the diffuser or air stone that is supplied with the ozone generator. However the drawback with this idea is that there is a risk of faeces contacting the diffuser. Then came the 'eureka' moment. A solution so simple and so obvious that I am at a loss to understand why it took me so long to think of it. Simply by wrapping the diffuser in soft toilet tissue paper, the diffuser stays clean and the paper can be thrown away after treatment. The toilet paper **must be** of the type that allows air to pass through.

Once you have created your wrapped diffuser it is a simple matter of placing it between your buttocks as near as possible to the area that is irritated.

Your buttocks will hold the diffuser in place allowing you to sit down whilst the ozone kills the microbes.

I presume that treatment times will be similar to those suggested for athlete's foot. I have only been able to try this out on a mild infection. A single treatment of 5 minutes brought about an almost immediate end to the itching.
I strongly recommend that you protect your seat with a sheet of polythene whilst carrying out the treatment. There are two reasons for this advice. The first is the simple fact that the polythene sheet will greatly assist in keeping the ozone where it is needed.
The second is to protect your seat. Ozone is destructive to some synthetic materials. Ozone can also bleach certain items. We have a mid-green bath mat with a light-green patch where it has been bleached as a result of coming into contact with ozone.

Just as I was preparing to publish this information I discovered yet another use for ozone, which I will share with you in the hopes that this may be of help to some of my readers, and because this snippet of information may not be available anywhere else.

I recently developed a split on the tip of one of my fingers, not for the first time, however this one not only failed to respond to my usual treatments, mainly consisting of softening creams, but also seemed to be getting deeper and was red, although not actually bleeding. It looked and felt sore, the slightest knock caused considerable pain. In desperation I decided to try ozone. One five minute treatment, mid evening, carried out by simply keeping the split directly in front of the short tube which projects from the ozone generator followed by a night's sleep led to a noticeable improvement by the following morning. The redness had gone and the split was less sensitive.

The following evening, by way of an insurance, I gave the split a second five minute treatment. Several days have now passed and the split has almost completely healed, despite the fact that, due to the lack of pain, I have forgotten to apply any softening cream.

For those of you who have read that ozone is actually bad for you. This is true in two scenarios. The first I have already cautioned you about, that is prolonged exposure to high concentrations of ozone. The second refers to bad ozone, that is the type of ozone which is created from pollutants, such as exhaust fumes in reaction with sunlight. This bad ozone can then be held at ground level, for example in smog, leading to people inhaling large and potentially dangerous amounts.

In reality the ozone that you will be generating to combat athlete's foot, when used sensibly, is unlikely to do any harm to the vast majority of users.
If ozone is used sensibly and carefully it should not be a cause for concern. Simply remember the golden rule and ensure adequate ventilation or air movement, especially if you have a lung problem.

I do not intend to expand on other uses for ozone as there is ample information available on the internet, suffice to say that once you have purchased your ozone generator you will no doubt discover multiple uses for it!

SOME ADDITIONAL FACTS ABOUT OZONE.

Your ozone generator works best with dry air. Elevated levels of atmospheric humidity will reduce the quantity of oxygen converted into ozone. The simplest solution in conditions of high humidity is to increase the treatment time.

Under normal conditions ozone returns to its previous state of oxygen in less than 60 minutes.
This is the reason why I have stated that you should not re-enter a room that has been sterilised for at least an hour after the end of the selected treatment time.

There is no known product more powerful than ozone for the sterilisation of air and surfaces. Ozone is unequalled in the speed with which it destroys harmful micro organisms.
Although ozone is also an effective water treatment product, I have not mentioned water here, as the equipment required is not a viable option in a domestic setting.

For those of you who own an in-ground swimming pool and want to go chlorine free, you will need to install a venturi plus an ozone generator of sufficient power for the size of your pool. It is also vital to eliminate all traces of chlorine before changing to ozone sterilisation as the combination of chlorine and ozone result in zero sterilisation, due to the fact that they cancel each other out. I recommend consulting a specialist on this subject before 'diving in at the deep end'.

The only 'nuisance' in a swimming pool that ozone is unable to kill is algae, therefore you will need to continue using an algicide.

In 1893 the first water treatment plant to use ozone was inaugurated. In 1906 an ozone treatment plant for drinking water was installed in Nice, France and is still in use.

In 1939 research proved that ozone can be used to prolong the storage life of fruit and vegetables.

In 1970 ozone began being used to treat bottled water.

OVERALL FOOT HEALTH.

For quite some time now I have been trying to figure out a way of treating the entirety of my feet with ozone. My feet had hard yellowish skin on parts of the soles, a tendency to splitting on the heels and had developed red blotches and patches of peeling skin, all of which caused me to feel somewhat embarrassed when wearing sandals during the summer months. The use of a polythene bag over my feet while treating athlete's foot had no effect on these unsightly blotches. I presumed that there were three possible reasons for the lack of a positive outcome.

The polythene bag may have prevented the ozone from contacting the entirety of my foot.
The quantity of ozone may have been insufficient or the treatment time was too short.
The unknown cause of the blotches may not respond to a treatment with ozone, although I considered it very likely that the condition may be related to athlete's foot and therefore I could see no reason why it should not respond to being treated with ozone.

Once I had purchased my 28 gph ozone generator, I came up with a plan. I felt that I needed a container with all of the following criteria;
It had to be large enough to contain both my foot and the ozone generator.

It had to be possible to form a seal around my leg to prevent the ozone from escaping, as it needed to provide a way of keeping as much of the ozone as possible within the container. **As previously stated, this high output type of ozone generator should only be used in a room that is unoccupied.**

There needed to be some way of 'suspending' my foot so that the ozone could make contact with the entirety of the foot being treated.

The rather clumsy, makeshift solution that I came up with was as follows. To make the container and the seal I employed a laundry basket which I placed inside a large polythene bin bag. Once the ozone generator and my foot were installed, I was able the wrap the open end of the bin bag around my leg and the mains lead. This I secured with a hook and loop ribbon.

It is absolutely vital to ensure that the polythene bag cannot contact the inlet of the generator. The ozone generator relies on a through-flow of air in order to prevent over-heating and to supply the oxygen required to convert into ozone. The laundry basket performs this function very well.

I am unable to think of a way of treating both feet at the same time due to the **essential requirement** of containing the ozone within the confines of the bag, other than having two of everything, one for each foot. Treating one foot at a time is obviously more time consuming, but as this treatment requires you to be seated, it can be carried out while doing something else. I could, for example, be treating one of my feet while sitting at my desk, writing this book.

The method that I used was to set the timer of the ozone generator to a slightly greater length of time than I felt that I required, so that I could make the seal around my leg **before** connecting the generator to the mains supply. I use an extension lead to simplify this operation, as once seated with your leg in place, your ability to move will be restricted.

If you decide to follow my example as outlined above, you will need to be aware that the level of ozone within the bag at the end of your selected treatment time will be dangerously high.
DO NOT ATTEMPT TO FOLLOW MY EXAMPLE UNLESS YOU CAN DO SO OUT OF DOORS

However the improvement in the appearance of my foot made all the effort worthwhile. A few days after my first ozone treatment there were visible signs that the blotches were fading and that the skin was starting to heal.

I have referred to my foot and not feet for a very good reason, in order to truly gauge the results I treated my left foot, keeping my right foot untreated in order that I could compare one against the other, making it easier to see the improvement.

A method of 'suspending' my foot during treatment required me to agitate the grey cells quite a bit. Surely there must be numerous ways of ensuring that the ozone can contact all of my foot! But what would actually be effective? In the end a rummage in my garage uncovered a plastic plant tray. The type of rather flimsy tray that holds 6 plants as a carry home pack, it has solid plastic sides and a lattice base. This was not very successful as it was inclined to crumple under the weight of my leg.

Another, stronger, contender for this task was a trivet as used for protecting surfaces from hot containers. Unfortunately the ozone attacked the steel core of the trivet despite having a protective layer of chrome plating, causing it to rust.
I now use a plastic lattice grill for the purpose. Materials that are resistant to ozone include silicone, stainless steel and some plastics. I am aware that one can buy a pot trivet made from silicone, this would be ideal.

Whatever you use, be sure to periodically move your foot slightly so that there are no areas that cannot be contacted by the ozone. For the same reason, spread and straighten your toes from time to time.

After 4 or 5 treatments, each of 10 minutes, I had a pleasant surprise.
I regularly soak my feet and whilst the skin is still soft, I remove as much of the hard skin as possible. Following the ozone treatments the hard skin on the foot that had been bathed in ozone was much easier than usual to remove with more dead skin than usual coming away.

The overall health of my left foot is greatly improved with a noticeable reduction in all of the symptoms previously mentioned.

ITCHING SCALP

I have experienced scalp irritation for more years than I care to remember. I was thinking that this irritation would be with me for the rest of my life, a thought that was reinforced by an elderly relative who also endured scalp irritation up until her death. Both of us had tried a variety of treatment shampoos with only temporary relief.

Since getting such good results treating athlete's foot with ozone, I had wondered if the ozone might possibly remedy an itching scalp. Even if that was a possibility, I was unable to envisage a method of keeping the ozone in place whilst at the same time avoiding the ozone from entering my nose during any potential treatment.

A disposable polythene shower cap seemed to be a likely contender with one drawback. Following my experience with an elastic band rapidly degrading when I used one to hold a polythene bag in place on my foot, I assumed that the same would happen to the elastic of a shower cap.

As my wife had a hotel shower cap, I decided to experiment. Much to my surprise the elastic did not degrade quite as quickly as I thought it might. It lasted for a single treatment of 15 minutes, after which the elastic was completely destroyed. I was content that it had lasted to the end of the treatment. After all, this type of shower cap costs as little as a few pennies to replace.

The next challenge was how to keep the silicone tube that conveys the ozone in place. After a couple of failed attempts, I came up with the following idea that worked even better than I had expected, although I felt that I looked ridiculous and as a result I locked myself in the room where I intended to carry out the treatment.

The method that worked for me was as follows. First I inserted the diffuser into the end of the flexible tubing. Using an old satin dressing gown tie, I loosely tied a single knot at the centre of the belt, I then passed the diffuser through the loose knot. Next I tightened the knot so that it gripped the flexible tubing at the point where the diffuser entered. I now placed the diffuser on top of my head, with the flexible tubing running down the back of my head and neck, and allowed the two ends of the dressing gown tie to fall down, one end on each side of my face. I now tied the two ends together under my chin, put on the shower cap and switched on the ozone generator. I was very surprised at how efficiently the shower cap kept the ozone in place, as I was completely unaware of the odour of ozone for the entire duration of the treatment.

When I removed the shower cap the odour of ozone was really quite strong, almost as if it had been concentrated. However, because the micro-organisms die very quickly when exposed to ozone, and because ozone returns to oxygen within a short period of time, there is no advantage in carrying the odour around with you for any more than 30 minutes.
After that you may very well want to shampoo your hair in order to wash away the odour.

I hope that you will be inspired by the treatments that I have developed and go on to develop your own. I can envisage, for example, that the treatment for jock itch could be easily adapted for treating an under-arm infection.

Therefore I am handing the baton to you so that you can proceed with your new-found tool that efficiently destroys fungal infections.

Other drug-free self-help health titles from the same author, available from Amazon.

COMMON COLD NO MORE.

A simple guide to reducing the symptoms of the common cold by as much as 99% without the use of drugs. The book explains in everyday language how you can reduce the symptoms of the common cold to a point where you may even forget that you have a cold, enabling you to completely avoid the painful infections that sometimes follow, such as congestion of the ears or sinuses which may ultimately require treatment with a course of antibiotics. It has taken me more than twenty years of trial and improvement to develop my system to the point that I can honestly state that it is possible to achieve up to a 99% reduction of the symptoms of the common cold, with complete recovery possible in less than a week. My method uses a readily available product, produced using two entirely natural ingredients, for as little as three days from the onset of a cold. I now feel fully confident about the effectiveness of my method and feel obliged to publish this information. You will need to purchase a 100% natural product, at a cost of around £30, which will treat 2 or 3 colds.

10 YEARS YOUNGER.

Learn how a little-known food supplement has improved my life and health in so many ways. At my current age of 72 I truly look and feel more like 62. This booklet is a completely independent and unbiased in-depth assessment of a food supplement. It describes many of the improved health benefits that I now experience on a daily basis. However, the improvements to my health are such that a review posted on their website would be far too long!! I am so delighted with the results that I now feel a moral obligation to make this information more widely available. I must point out that I do not receive any financial gain from the producer of this supplement. Producers of supplements are not legally allowed to state the benefits of their products, whereas I, as an individual, can inform you of the health benefits that I currently enjoy.

Some of these improvements include:

greater stamina.

improved skin condition and hair colour.

general feeling of well-being.

increased mental ability.

The supplement has eliminated pains in my upper leg muscles and back which were previously constant but getting worse with each passing year.

Even my reduction in height, due to ageing, has been reversed.

My book lists many of the benefits that I currently enjoy and names the all-important wholly natural supplement.

Please note that this supplement is NOT an overnight or miracle cure as most of the benefits took between 3 and 9 months to become evident. It has to be stated that any supplement can, at best, only provide one's body with the elements that it needs to repair itself.

I have left you some space to keep a record of your progress.
Notes

Notes

Notes

Notes

Notes